STANDING TALL
Twenty-One Days In May

JACQUI TAM

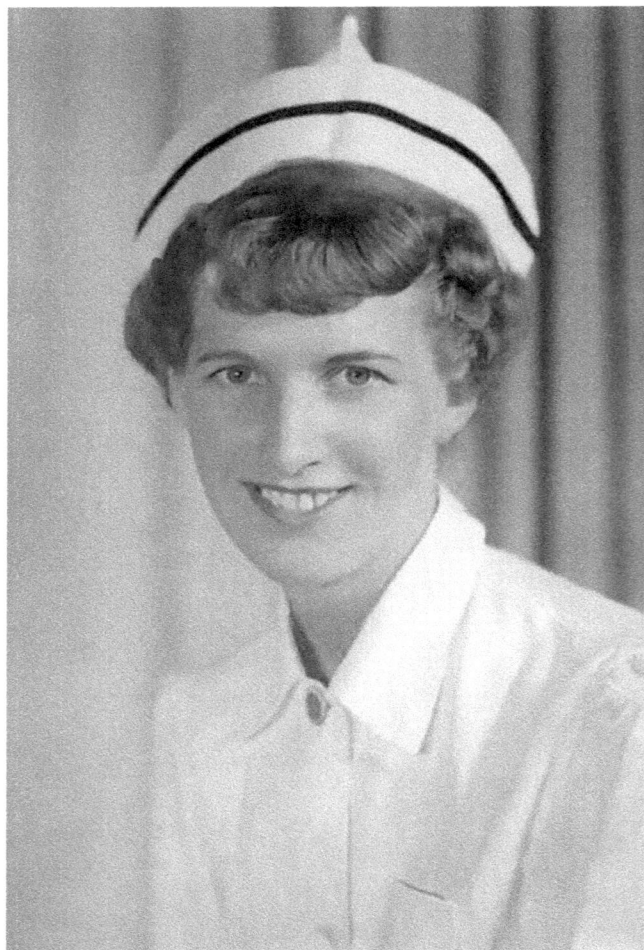

STANDING TALL
Twenty-One Days In May

JACQUI TAM

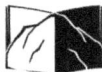

ICEBERG

Published in Canada by Iceberg Publishing, Edmonton

Library and Archives Canada Cataloguing in Publication
Tam, Jacqui, 1960-, author
    Twenty-one days in May : standing tall / Jacqui Tam.
ISBN 978-1-926817-75-0 (paperback)
    1. Tam, Jacqui, 1960-. 2. Cancer--Patients--Family
relationships--Newfoundland and Labrador. 3. Mothers
and
daughters--Canada--Biography. 4. Children of cancer
patients--Canada--Biography. I. Title. II. Title: 21 days in
May.
RC265.6.B37T34 2016   362.19699'40092   C2016-
905886-7

First ebook edition: September 2016
First print edition: September 2016

Cover Design: Kenneth Tam

Cover Photo: Signal Hill in St. John's, Newfoundland.

ICEBERG PUBLISHING
9218-319 Ellerslie Road SW
Edmonton AB Canada T6X OK6
icebergpublishing.com

For my mother and friend,
Mary Louise Barron.

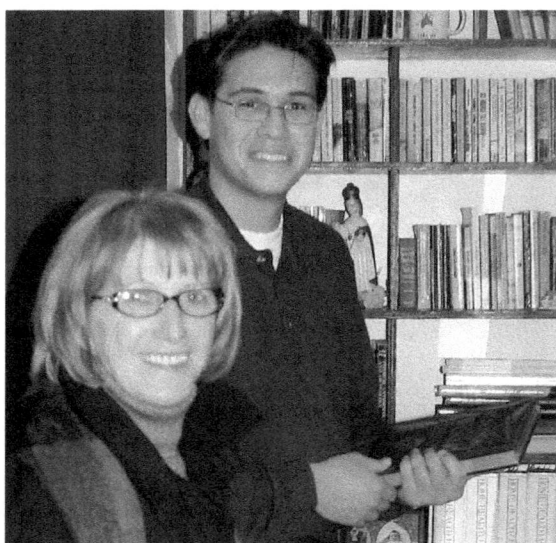

Foreword

By Kenneth Tam

When my mother handed me this manuscript, she had only one question: *Is it worth publishing?*

It was an honest question, rooted in a concern that I understood. Unlike *A Daughter's Gift*, the seminal and now award-winning memoir that was the genesis of Iceberg Publishing — and which taught me how to write — this story comes from a different place. Instead of crossing time and space, it holds its counsel within a three-week window. Though it touches on the certainties of my mother's relationship with my grandmother, it is rooted in the daily reality of a proud woman and her daughter, quietly approaching an end neither is naïve about.

The differences between this story and *A Daughter's Gift* were inevitable. My grandmother's death affected my mother very differently than my grandfather's had.

This was not just because the circumstances were so distinct — abrupt and unexpected, instead of protracted and inevitable — but because Jacqui Tam's relationship with Mary Louise Barron was truly different than her relationship with Richard Joseph Barron.

So much of what my mother holds dearest and consciously chooses to be part of her identity came from my grandfather's quiet strength and trust. He gave her courage and belief in herself, as any father should do — must do — for his children. He was her rock and inspiration. Mary Barron was her drive.

My grandmother was the sort of nurse who would see darkness, and move towards it. Her calling was to help those in pain, and that dedication shaped both the way she treated others, and the expectations she placed on her daughter.

She always impressed upon my mother the need for steel, determination, and toughness, but also kindness. She expected her only daughter to set the same example that she herself strived to embody. She gave her daughter love, but she tested her always. This was, I think, as important to my mother's life, and my life, and even to the creation of Iceberg Publishing, as everything my grandfather shared with us.

But it wasn't easy. And it's an almost impossible story to tell.

So instead of trying to capture it all, my mother has chosen this final chapter — this fragment that brings everything that mattered between her and her mother into sharp focus. Paired with *A Daughter's Gift,* these twenty-one days will show you how two so very different parents together managed to forge one of the most formidable people I know.

As a son, I am forever proud of my mother. This book is yet another reason why.

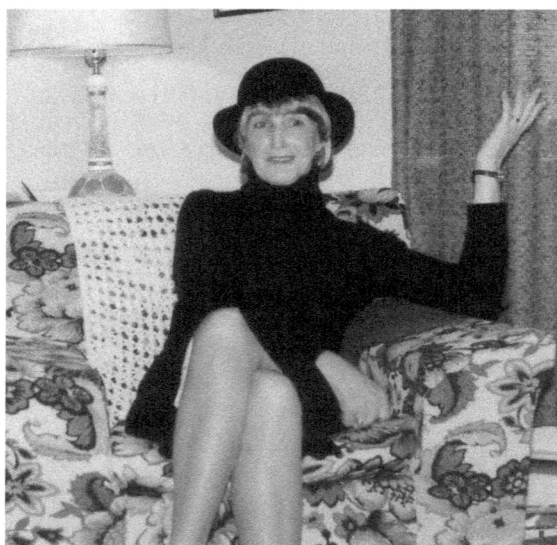

Prologue

Words are such powerful things.   Right words...
wrong words... unspoken words. Words we never have
the chance to say. Words we wish we'd never uttered.

The last thing I have ever wanted to do, with my
words, is to damage a treasured relationship.

The last thing I wanted to do when I wrote a book
about my father, our relationship, and the heartbreaking
journey that is Alzheimer's, was to hurt my mother. I
didn't want her to feel that I had somehow betrayed
her, or shared moments too private to ever be shared.
But I knew there were sections of the book that would
potentially do just that, and I feared their impact even
though I knew there was no other way to tell the story.

I was so concerned she'd be upset that immediately
after I packaged up a copy of the manuscript and
couriered it to her in Newfoundland from my then-home

in southern Alberta, I took my own copy and marked with yellow sticky notes every paragraph I thought might upset her. Then I counted the days until she would have received and read it, and waited for the telephone to ring.

I stood leaning against the kitchen counter in my home when I answered her call, my gaze directed towards the window that looked out onto our deck and the farmer's field beyond. The manuscript with sticky notes was on the counter beside me, though I had no idea what I could say about it if she challenged my memories of how she had been.

As soon as she spoke, I could hear the tears in her eyes... they were in her voice as well.

I was really like that, wasn't I? she asked.

Yes, was my quiet reply.

Don't change a word, through the tears, her conviction was firm. *Not a single word. People need to know. People need to know that's what Alzheimer's does to the loved ones. People need to know...*

I had not expected that. Perhaps I should have, but I had doubted that my mother would be willing to let others know how much pain she had suffered, and how that pain had affected our lives.

Despite being outgoing, Mary Louise Barron was an intensely private person. Her role in my father's story was one of intense devotion and love, but the experience of caring for him ravaged her and left scars that never healed even though she hid them well. In *A Daughter's Gift*, I wrote about the changes as I had witnessed them — talked of depression and anger and many other things. I had relayed some of the most intimate and heartbreaking moments of my father's later years — moments that had caused all of us incredible anguish.

But despite the pain she felt reading the manuscript, and despite its honest account of her suffering, she didn't ask me to change a word.

Not a single word.

That she didn't ask me to hide her suffering because she believed its truth could help others was, I thought then, everything that needed to be said about her courage, about her character, about the measure of this extraordinary woman.

But I was wrong.

There is more to be said. There is more to be

remembered, in love, about the woman who will be with me always.

The Days After and Before

On the morning of my 46th birthday, I awoke in a hotel room, my husband at my side. There are sometimes moments between sleep and wakefulness when whatever may have been haunting you the night before is suspended… forgotten. When you can simply appreciate the first moments of consciousness without any sense of what has passed or what is to come.

Not on this particular morning.

Peter may have already been awake, or he may have woken when he heard me stir. I don't recall. He wished me happy birthday, kissed me gently, and then quietly got out of bed, pulled on pants and a shirt, and went to the front lobby for a newspaper.

I stayed in bed, waiting.

He returned to the room a few minutes later, silently handed me the folded pages. *Yes, it's there,* was his response to my unspoken query. Dread mixed with anticipation and a feeling of disconnected realities as I opened the paper, then turned to the obituaries and scanned for my mother's name. Began to read.

On May 27th, 2006, the morning of my 46th birthday, in a hotel room in St. John's, Newfoundland, the beloved city of my birth, I read my mother's obituary. Unbelievable, inconceivable, and yet somehow inevitable.

When I pushed the hotel bed linens aside, shivering even though it wasn't cold, I consciously reached to the back of my mind for the image and the sound of my mother struggling for her last breaths just two days before.

I ignored my memory of the silence that had followed in the private Intensive Care room... the sudden emptiness of her always so vibrant body. I thought instead of the people I had not yet been able to reach with the news, who would be reading the paper this morning and sitting, grief-stricken in their chairs. I silently rehearsed the story of twenty-one days in May, getting ready to tell it as often as it needed to be told, to all those who would be gathering in disbelief and grief. And I prepared to wrap myself in the safety of an outfit my mother would have liked, so I would be the daughter she could be proud of as I helped to give her a fitting farewell.

The story of those twenty-one days is neither unique nor unusual. Few stories truly are. As much pain or shock or loss as one family is experiencing at any given time, other families are going through so much worse. But my family and my mother's many friends somehow thought she would live forever, or at least for as long as anyone else who needed her was alive.

The thought that she had been incapable of rallying against the fluid buildup in her lungs after surgery, dying just twenty-one days after her cancer diagnosis, seemed impossible. But it wasn't impossible; it was real. And the fact that we would be gathering at a funeral home in just a few hours, in a room that would undoubtedly be filled with flowers, was a stark reminder of that.

If you have previously read *A Daughter's Gift*, you will know already that flowers — roses and stargazer lilies especially — have immense meaning in my life beyond what would sound logical. Pink roses assured us that the bone cancer I had been diagnosed with was not bone cancer at all. A red rose carried the message that my father would be fine, despite his lung cancer diagnosis.

And beautiful stargazer lilies connected my father with me across time, space, and the incredible loss that is Alzheimer's.

But in *A Daughter's Gift*, I did not share the story of my mother and her older sister, Lillian. I remember Aunt Lillian as a tall, regal woman who suffered greatly with arthritis, migraines, and as time went on, a myriad of other health problems. She lived with her husband and five children in the heart of St. John's, in a stately home with high ceilings, a tall staircase, and no front yard. As much as anyone, she was one of the reasons I existed — her then-boyfriend Vince had introduced my father to my mother when she was bedridden with tuberculosis.

My mother and Lillian were extremely close — much closer than I ever realized as a child. Lillian was sister and friend, and almost a second mother as well. As they both aged, and as it became increasingly likely that one of the illnesses my aunt was fighting would claim her, the two sisters made a pact. Whoever died first, they agreed, would send the other sister a sign to prove there was more to existence than this one life, and reassure her that she'd arrived in another place happy and all was well. They would tell no one about the pact — they could only trust the sign when it appeared if no one else ever knew of their promises.

I have no idea how long after that conversation Aunt Lillian died, though I do know it was much sooner than either of them would have hoped. I also know that it was still in the period before my father's death, when I would attend funerals only if I had absolutely no other choice. In those times, I avoided funeral homes and wakes at all cost — I could not bear the sight of death.

It was out of character for me, then, to be so determined to not only attend Lillian's wake, but to arrive at the funeral home as soon as it opened on the first morning. Surprised, but willing to go along with the feeling that I was doing what I needed to do, I cleared the hour between 10 and 11 a.m. in my schedule, and left my office to go to the florist in the shopping mall across the street. Convention under these circumstances would have been to order flowers and have them delivered, but the same strange conviction insisted that I bring them with me.

The discussion with the lady in the flower shop should have been unremarkable as I tried to figure out what I wanted to order, but when I finally decided on a half-dozen white roses, she told me that I'd have to wait for the florist to get them ready. The arrangement therefore couldn't be prepared until early that afternoon, at which point it could be delivered direct to the funeral home.

But I have to bring something with me, I told her. *I have to.* She tried to convince me that the delivery would be fine — better in fact, and normal.

She was right. The logical thing would have been to leave for the funeral home, knowing the flowers would follow. But I couldn't. I knew I simply couldn't walk into the wake empty-handed.

So I thought for a moment before shrugging my shoulders: *Ok then, just give me one white rose. Yes, that would be perfect, just one white rose. Wrapped in paper. And the half-dozen can come later.*

Tears filled my mother's eyes when I walked into the funeral home a short time later, holding what she recognized immediately as a flower wrapped in paper.

You brought it, she said. *You brought one white rose, didn't you?*

Aunt Lillian's sign. She had promised she would send one white rose. And I delivered it for her.

Time stands still, just for an instant, in moments like that.

My mother never doubted that the rose I placed in her outstretched hands was from her sister, and I never doubted that my aunt had somehow compelled me to deliver it for her. Why else would I have been so determined? There could be no other explanation for insisting I had to bring something so specific to a place I would never normally have gone.

Aunt Lillian had promised my mother a rose, a white rose, and she didn't waste any time sending it.

After this, it was inevitable that, on what we both knew would be her last morning, I would ask my mother if she would send me a sign. She had refused any additional medical intervention, and we knew her time would be measured in hours. Speaking was torture for her, and I regretted not having had the courage to raise this question earlier, but I leaned over her bed anyway and asked whether there was a sign I should look for… a sign like the one Lillian had sent her… one that would let me know she was with my father and all was well.

Pulling her oxygen mask away, she held up the index finger on her left hand, and struggled for an instant to gather enough air.

One red rose.

A pause, her finger moving back and then forward again

And one white.

Her voice was like gravel.

One red rose, and one white? I wanted to be sure.

One red rose, and one white. She confirmed with a nod, before my hand and hers returned the oxygen mask to her face.

One red rose, and one white. Aunt Lillian's white rose, my father's red. Together. This was my mother's sign.

Others came after she told me this — the steady parade of people she wanted to see, making their way to her bedside. I slipped out to the soft lights of the private waiting room that sheltered families who were coming to terms with the truth that there would be one fewer member when they left the hospital.

I told the aunts who were gathered that she'd told me what to look for, that there would be a sign. But I would not tell them what it was. I would only tell them after I'd seen it, not before.

I was not thinking of any of this that morning in my hotel room, though. I did not think of signs. I did not look for roses or wonder where or when or if I'd see them. Instead, I wrapped myself in the protection of appearances, coping beneath the armor of a black suit that my mother would have thought appropriate.

Peter and I arrived at the funeral home before anyone else so we'd have time to ensure everything was as it should be... entered the room and moved to stand beside my mother's casket. She rested there, the mother of my memory, in her white nurse's uniform and navy blue cape. But things weren't quite right: her instructions had been very precise — she had wanted her Registered Nurse's cap, with its black band striking against the white, beside her in the casket but not on her head. They had affixed it to her head, leaving us with the decision as to whether or not we should risk removing it — messing the carefully arranged hair — or leave it in place. But she had wanted it off, so we removed it.

Such small things become so important in moments like those. You drink them in — lock them, and the emotions that go with them, into your mind and heart. Then, as you begin to absorb everything around you, you start to consciously register details that had previously gone unnoticed.

It strikes me as odd, in retrospect, that as important as the flowers on my father's casket had been, I barely noticed the ones on my mother's. I cannot recall the arrangements, or even the process of choosing them. But I suddenly noticed the room was overflowing with them. They were everywhere.

As I turned my back on my mother, of course my eyes were drawn to one particular arrangement: lilies, carnations, other flowers I don't recall... and in the midst of them all, one single red rose, and one white.

A physical jolt. Part joy, part agony. Profound and intense.

That's her sign, I told Peter. *This is what she told me to look for.*

When I read the card, my eyes filled with tears: the flowers were from Esther and Jeanie Buckley. Just as I was the right person to bring Lillian's rose to my mother, Esther was the only person who could have sent my Mom's roses to me. Thirty-two years prior, when I was fourteen and facing a bone cancer diagnosis, she was the dear friend who had first given us reason to understand that roses were messages.

Then, the roses had come to tell us that I was, unbelievably, cancer-free. Now, they came to tell me that my mother and father were reunited, and that all was truly well.

For the next two hours, while talking with the family and friends who came to pay their respects, I watched the door for Esther and her sister Jeanie. When they arrived, I excused myself and went to them immediately. I brought Esther to the arrangement, I told her about my mother's sign, and I thanked her. For the second time in my life, she had made possible a message that was beyond logic and reason — a message that mattered so much.

For after three heartbreaking weeks that somehow captured everything I understood about her and our relationship, my mother had sent me the sign that all was well.

Day 1
Friday, May 5

It was a Friday when my mother called — about 3:00 in the afternoon.

Normally, I would have been at my office at Wilfrid Laurier University, in Waterloo, Ontario. However, this was my first week back to work after having had surgery, and I was still much more tired that I expected to be. So I'd packed my briefcase at noon and gone home to sleep.

Mom and I had been talking two, three, four times a day that month — my surgery had been without complications of either the immediate or long-term type, but she needed to know how I was recovering, and I needed to hear her continuing reassurances. We had not connected on the previous day, though — I was on the mend and it was simply a break for both of us. Or so I'd thought.

She asked first how I was feeling, and I explained

that I was doing okay — that I'd just come home early to sleep. She asked next after Atlas, our much-loved German Shepherd who had been diagnosed with lymphoma on February 15th, and who was fighting a valiant battle.

Then she said: *I have news, but I don't want you to be upset.*

A pause came next — a pause that in hindsight seems the type that was meant to give me the slightest warning that everything was about to change forever. I don't know if I said anything after she spoke. I remember only the pause, and the three words that followed.

I have cancer.

The rest came out in a rush. A trip to the family doctor the day before to have what she suspected was a hernia in her right lower abdomen checked... an immediate call from that doctor to a specialist... a CT scan that same afternoon... a visit with the specialist the following day — this first day. The diagnosis.

I imagined what it was like for my mother to receive such news alone. I pictured her in the clinical setting — always so terrifying for me, always so comfortable for her — and felt her isolation acutely, even though she probably preferred that there were no witnesses to her reaction.

I couldn't help but wonder how she had felt as she walked to her car in the hospital parking lot. How she managed to drive home — alone — with the knowledge she now carried. What she did in the minutes and hours before she picked up the phone to start making phone calls.

I wondered all those things, but as was her way, she was already offering only the information she wanted me to have.

I have surgery next week, and then I'll have treatment if needed, she continued in a rush. *Chemotherapy. It's just one tumor, so they'll get it all. And I'm still coming to Kenneth's graduation in June. I'll be well enough by then. I'll probably have lost my hair but I'll get a wig.*

One should feel something sharp at moments like this; I felt only numbness. One should probably cry, like I did when I had called her to tell her about Atlas's diagnosis. But my eyes remained completely dry.

She sounded strong, and in absolute control — as always. Her weekend was all planned out: she'd be cleaning windows and curtains. I was her daughter, so she needed just as much control from me. At least that's what I think she needed. Because I had learned such control from her, and now it was what I could give back.

I don't know what my next words were. I don't know how long the call lasted. But as we said our goodbyes, I remembered distinctly what she had said to me a few weeks earlier, when the doctor had told me my ovarian cyst had been benign. That I didn't have cancer.

Cancer, she had said, *that one word changes everything, doesn't it?*

Yes, I was thinking, *it changes everything.*

When our call was over, I stayed sitting on the step until my then twenty-one-year-old son Kenneth arrived to check on me, and to ask why I hadn't moved after the call had obviously ended.

That was Mary, I told him. *She had news.*

But she doesn't want us to be upset.

Day 2
Saturday, May 6

My mother returned to work as a nurse when I was two-years-old. My paternal grandmother — Nan Barron — had come to live with us. She would be able to care for me and my brothers, Steve and Rik, who were eight and five respectively, while my mother was at the hospital.

My mother's Monday to Friday work schedule meant that housework as well as other chores and errands mostly had to be tackled on the weekend. Laundry usually got started on Friday night. In the early days that meant hours spent running clothes through the now antique wringer washer that was set up in our basement, where rows of lines had also been installed so clothes could be hung to dry. Housework was usually done on Saturday morning, and through as much of the afternoon as was needed. Sunday morning, after church, there was the ironing, while the Sunday dinner cooked.

Our treat, as I grew older and we were able to get all or most of the housework done on Friday evening, was to go to the Avalon Mall to browse. Always in the morning (because we didn't like the afternoon crowds), we'd visit our favorite stores, hunt for bargains, study the latest styles, and then treat ourselves to lunch in the Mall's tiny café. I'd have a small plate of French fries and a soft drink. My mother would usually have a bran muffin and coffee, and one or two of my fries. I'd watch as she reapplied her lipstick after we'd finished.

If we knew we still had housework to do when we got home, that fact would hang over us. Still having the housework to do ruined the morning, my mother always said.

Decades later, this pattern of activity still guides my weekends. Housework and errands are mostly reserved for Friday night, Saturday, and Sunday. Saturday morning shopping — before the crowds — is still a treat. And if housework still needs to be done when we get home, that continues to hang over me... not as strongly as it once did, but there nonetheless.

On this particular Saturday morning — May 6th, 2006 — I found a strange comfort in the routine of housework. In that routine, I could find a modicum of control in a world that had fundamentally shifted.

Peter hadn't been home when my mother had called the previous afternoon, because he had been in Toronto refereeing at a squash tournament. We expected him home sometime between 10:30 p.m. and midnight, and Kenneth and I agreed to wait until then to give him the news. Navigating Highway 401 between Toronto and Waterloo was challenging enough; there was nothing to be gained by distracting him with such news.

In the meantime, Kenneth and I had discussed the few details my mother had provided. The single tumor was in her lower stomach, and she was having surgery on Thursday, May 11th. From what she said the cancer was localized, but they would likely do chemotherapy to ensure no other traces remained. And she would still travel to Waterloo in the first week of June, for his graduation from university.

We both knew, of course, that the twenty-four hour turnaround between the appointment with her family doctor and the booking of surgery meant there was a great deal to be concerned about. The system only moves that quickly when it is imperative that it do so, and sometimes not even then. But some truths are best not spoken.

That night, our telephone was busy. I made calls to my mother, who took them while sitting in the chair she always occupied when talking on the phone — the chair at the heart of the house she'd lived in for more than forty years. I spoke to my brother Steve, who lived just outside Vancouver. To other people I've since forgotten.

We checked my office schedule for the coming weeks. We checked flight schedules. I would go to St. John's to be with her for the surgery, of course. Steve, who would know how best to care for a post-op patient at home, would arrive about a week later, when she could expect to be discharged from hospital. Kenneth decided he would travel with me — so soon after my surgery, I wasn't quite ready to handle luggage on my own, but more than that, he would not send me to face this alone. Peter needed to stay at home with Atlas to manage his cancer treatments, but he'd come later if he had to.

And so on Saturday, in addition to the regular, now comforting chores, we booked relatively convenient mid-morning flights out of Toronto that would see us arriving in St. John's late in the afternoon of the day before my mother's surgery.

I started an inventory of my wardrobe, sorting through clothes that would be appropriate for the hospital so I could determine if I needed to sew anything before we left. I checked in regularly with the woman who had decided that, in addition to her own regular housework, it was time to wash her curtains. I heard the sense of purpose and direction in her voice. I marveled at how that voice could be so strong and calm — happy even.

But I'd grown up with my mother. We knew each other well. I understood why the last thing she would do on that particular weekend was let things slide. I understood what her purpose was and exactly why she was cleaning the curtains.

And happiness didn't even enter the equation.

Day 3
Sunday, May 7

With newly laundered curtains reinstalled and smelling fresh from their hastily-planned spring cleaning, my mother tackled her closets on the second day after her diagnosis. This even though I didn't recall them being particularly disorganized or messy on my previous visit.

Through all the years of my childhood, the closet in my parents' room had always been neatly organized — my mother's clothing taking about two-thirds of the space, my father's the rest. In the years that had passed since my brothers and I had permanently moved out of the house, the closets in our rooms had provided additional space for my mother to utilize. My dad's passing had further lightened the burden, and over the years, off-season wardrobes and clothing that wasn't yet ready to be passed along had been allocated to new locations.

Coats. Hats. Shoes. Bits and pieces that needed a

home. This Sunday wasn't about cleaning, it was about bringing further order to contents most people would have already thought totally organized.

A few days after this, I would have reason to question whether the impression my mother had given me of her activity-filled weekend had been accurate — even for the young and healthy, cleaning curtains and organizing closets can be tiring. But on that Sunday, I heard only confidence and strength in her voice when she explained her purpose, and I believed what she told me. Or perhaps I chose to believe, knowing that was the role we both needed me to play.

In my own home some 3,000 kilometres away, I sorted through my closet to find the right outfit for traveling. The right outfit to wear when taking her to the hospital. The right outfits for hours or days with her at the hospital. The right outfit to wear when bringing her home. If you did not know my mother and her attention to appearance, this particular focus might seem out of place under the circumstances. But in my mother's presence, the right clothing for the right occasion was essential. At all times, and especially in times of extreme stress, standards had to be maintained.

But my selection came up short. I was well equipped to deal with my regular needs — I had a healthy selection of business clothes and some casual wear for the weekend. But neither would suffice in the circumstances.

So while my mother cleaned closets, I searched through my fabric stash and patterns, and began to sew — black wool bootleg trousers, and a black-on-black print poncho out of a heavy brocade-like fabric.

I could wrap myself in the poncho, I thought. Sitting in the vinyl covered chairs of hospital waiting rooms, I could at least wrap myself in fabric I loved.

Day 4
Monday, May 8

The thing about the kind of news my mother received on Friday, May 5th is that it completely changes everything. There is no part of life that isn't impacted — even the small things, like how to answer the inevitable Monday morning query about your weekend.

I remember no specifics about returning to work that Monday morning. I'm sure I shared the information with whoever was necessary... made arrangements to take time off again beginning on Wednesday... began the process of organizing files and sorting out the deadlines I would not be able to change.

There were also logistical challenges. My mother didn't own a computer. We'd wanted to get one for her, or at least give her one of ours that was being retired, thinking she'd enjoy email and the internet, but she was never interested in entering that world. Her preferred communications methods were telephone and face-to-face, so her home had none of the technologies that would be necessities for us as we stayed in touch with my office, or prepared the summer releases for Iceberg Publishing — the company Peter, Kenneth and I had established four years before.

We'd therefore need to stay in a hotel where we'd have internet access, and where my mother would have no reason to feel guilty for keeping us from our work. She would also be under no pressure to prepare meals or provide clean sheets and linens, and she wouldn't have the stress of us suggesting we do those things for her. Most importantly, I would realize after I arrived, there would be no need for her to keep up appearances — she wouldn't have to pretend to be feeling stronger, better than she was.

But to be completely honest, there was another reason I don't think I could have handled staying in my childhood home on this particular trip. Returning to 37 Penetanguishene after my father died and we'd moved away had grown more difficult with every trip back. It was as if the very floors and walls were imbued with a deep regret and pain. On rare occasions I could feel my father's presence; most of the time it seemed that nothing of his spirit remained. In the house, I felt a deep sadness.

The house didn't remind me of all that had been wonderful about my childhood, and there had been much. It reminded me of loss, and emptiness, and lives grown smaller as time moved on. Best not to try to deal with those emotions and everything else as well. Best to find an escape.

And so a hotel was booked — the hotel that became something of a second home, with my cousin Nikki at the front desk, the best hot turkey sandwich (Newfoundland style) on the room service menu, a view of St. John's Harbour and Signal Hill, and the kindest staff you could hope to meet.

Then, on Monday evening, before one more day at the office and my final packing, we celebrated Mother's Day in my house. I have never liked to celebrate special occasions before they arrive. It seems a tempting of fate and I carry enough of the superstitious Irish heritage to make me fear a jinx — as if the fates are watching for one slip-up, where they can catch you and pounce, blurt *I'll show you*, and ensure the day being celebrated early never arrives.

But in 2006 we made an exception — we changed the date and I had my own personal Mother's Day celebration.

Atlas, in another stage of treatment for his aggressive cancer, sat smiling by my chair in his usual spot. I can hear his breathing even now. I can see his large smile, and the eyes that somehow put laughter and joy before the pain that would have been his constant companion. There were gifts, including an iPod because I would need music for writing, for calming, for intermittent escapes.

It was good that I had it.

Day 5
Tuesday, May 9

I sometimes think that packing for trips would be so much less complicated if the trips themselves were uncomplicated, or if they were for the single and simple purpose of enjoyment. If you didn't have to worry about what or who you were leaving behind, or what you needed to bring 'in case', or what you would face while away. I can't remember the number of times I've packed for trips, but there have been relatively few times that the packing has been truly uncomplicated.

May 9th was not an uncomplicated packing experience. Every outfit worn in my mother's presence would be assessed, head to toe. My mother's sense of style was impeccable, and it was impossible for her to look at her daughter without taking stock and determining if she approved of the choices made. I didn't want to let her down, especially not under these circumstances.

In the hours available to me between Friday afternoon and Tuesday night, after I'd completed all the other tasks that needed doing prior to the trip, I'd spent sufficient time at the sewing machine to add the new items that could be combined with existing clothes to provide outfits for the anticipated number of days and situations. And so I began laying out everything on the bed, 'visiting the house' clothes... 'hotel room' clothes... 'hospital' clothes...

Everything was planned as carefully as possible. And yet I agonized.

Then there were the required files from work — human resource challenges being dealt with, communications plans around the issues and initiatives of the day, projects that had already suffered from the three weeks I'd been missing for my surgery, and three Iceberg Publishing titles in various stages of preparation for release in July.

Three books for the summer later became standard for us, but this was the first time we would be attempting that many — the fifth book in the *Equations* series, and the first two books in an entirely new series called *Defense Command*. Editing still needed to be done, so hundreds of pages were packed into various suitcases. There were questions about how to bring along electronic files — we hadn't had to travel with those before. Two laptops, hundreds of pages, and an iPod that would serve as an external hard drive — everything essential from our two offices was traveling with us.

In the years since, we've turned traveling with manuscripts, books, and event displays and supplies into something of an art form, but at that time, it was still fairly new to us. Systems that later served us so well were still in the process of being developed.

It's interesting as I write this; I feel like I did when I was packing that night. Not quite going around in circles, but *almost* — and experiencing that same anxiousness in the pit of my stomach, a fear that I'm somehow not going to make it work. Like those bad dreams where you're convinced you'll never actually complete a task, or reach your destination… or that you will arrive, but everything you need will be somewhere else. Or you'll be in your pajamas.

I was haunted, too, by questions of whether I'd be able to cope with what I was soon to face. Honestly, I questioned everything. And then I got angry with myself, because packing was so much easier than what my mother was facing.

Eventually all the suitcases, briefcases and other carry-ons were filled. Eventually, I slept. A troubled, heartsick sleep.

Because while I was not alone in my home, my mother was alone in hers. Totally and completely, except for her fears and her courage, and feelings she would never share.

Day 6
Wednesday, May 10

We were in the air when my mother underwent a colonoscopy that caused her doctor to shake his head in puzzlement and make the decision to delay her surgery. He had expected to find the cancer in her colon, but didn't. Deciding then that the problem must have been in her uterus, he advised a delay so he could have a surgeon more experienced in that area join him. My brother Rik had driven her to and from that appointment; we would take a taxi from the airport to her house when we arrived, so we could see her before retrieving her car for our stay. She wouldn't be using it, after all.

In all the times I'd flown into that particular airport, this made for a strange first. In St. John's, only business travelers from elsewhere usually have no one to meet them at the airport; if family or friends lived even remotely nearby, you could always bank on being picked up. It was tradition to find a small crowd watching as the plane disembarked, waiting to welcome people home — because even if they lived away, Newfoundland was still and always would be *home*.

So there seemed a particular significance to knowing that on this occasion my mother would not be waiting at the entrance to the baggage area — that instead she was at home, watching the time but waiting for us to come to her.

The afternoon was sunny and the temperature pleasant when the taxi dropped us off and unloaded our luggage onto the paved driveway. There was no need to bring the suitcases inside since we'd be moving them into my mother's car for the journey to the hotel, so instead we left them there and approached the back door. My mother was not by the door as I expected her to be — *she must not have heard the taxi arrive,* I remember thinking — but the door was unlocked, so we let ourselves in.

The ranch style house I grew up in has two front doors, one of which we called the back door. The back door was driveway level and immediately to the right of the large garage door; it was the everyday entrance for family members and friends. The front door was situated up a short flight of stairs roughly in the centre of the house between two large windows; it was reserved for special occasions and guests.

This back door was added along with the garage after the house had been built. When you entered, there were doors to the garage on the left, and a flight of stairs going up what would have originally been the outside of the house on the right. The door at the top entered immediately into the kitchen, and in addition to room on the landing for coats and shoes, the area provided space for a refrigerator that had, when I was a child, been much smaller and in the kitchen.

My mother was standing in the kitchen doorway at the top of the stairs. I have no memory of what she was wearing, or even her expression. What was so striking was the fact that while she had obviously heard us arrive, she had stayed at the top of the stairs instead of coming down to greet us.

The next realization was how desperately thin she was. My mother had vowed as a young woman that she would never succumb to what was at the time known as 'middle-age spread'. She may not have agreed, but those who knew her would have said she was most successful in that regard — trim and attractive always. However, on Wednesday, May 10th, I suddenly realized that when she'd happily told me a couple of weeks before that she'd *lost a little weight*, she had in fact been managing my expectations.

She'd said she was about 130 pounds. If she was 100, that's as much as she could be. And the doorframe was holding her up as surely as it held the door itself.

Communication is as much about what is not spoken as what is spoken. I did not tell her how thin she looked; I did not need to. I did not remark on how fragile she felt when I hugged her. Again, I did not need to. Instead she explained that the surgery had been delayed, and that it was good news because it meant we had time to do some things together that we wouldn't otherwise have done.

And, as I think we both knew in that moment and on that day, we would never do again.

Day 7
Thursday, May 11

They say memories are stored safely in our brains, that even when we cannot remember specifics, they somehow still exist. I don't know if that's true. I just know that I don't remember the specifics of the afternoon of Wednesday, May 10th in any great detail.

We arrived at my mother's house and quickly adjusted to the revised schedule for the week that would follow. We left for the hotel, checked in, navigated the unfamiliar but thankfully small car into the underground parking lot, rode the elevator to our room, and began the process that turned the room with two double beds temporarily into our own personal space.

We'd buy our supply of breakfast and snack foods and bottled water later, but placing our manuscripts on the desk, shoes along the wall, toiletries in the bathroom, and clothes in the closet, achieved the very necessary goal of making the space feel a little less impersonal and a little more like ours. Kenneth and I were alike in that regard: our first task in any hotel room was to make it somehow ours. Then we returned to 37 Penetanguishene at the appointed time, to pick up my mother and take her for a pizza supper at the same restaurant we'd visited together on our last trip home.

I'd realized how thin she was when I saw her earlier in the afternoon. What I hadn't realized, because she hadn't moved from her station in the doorway, was that thin also meant frail. Even in the most difficult periods of her life, even at her thinnest, she would never have been called frail. Even when sick with pneumonia, or suffering from intense vertigo, or beyond exhausted while caring for my father during his decade-long struggle with Alzheimer's, there was a core strength that somehow superseded the illness or the fatigue.

Had she not been so intensely focused on keeping her footing, I'm sure she would have recognized my shock when I first saw how gingerly and slowly she moved down the stairs, and out into the driveway. Just as I'm sure I would have seen her discomfort when she realized her difficulties were being witnessed. But her eyes were cast downward, and by the time she looked up again, my expression was schooled. As was hers.

I don't actually recall if I was ever told about the importance of maintaining appearances when growing up, but there is no doubt it's a lesson I learned as I watched my mother through the years and learned to model my behaviors after hers. No matter the grief, no matter the pain, it was important that the appearance of calm and strength be maintained.

My mother was clearly in pain that evening. Intense pain. Indeed, every action seemed to require extreme concentration, including the simple movement of fork to mouth. Still she smiled. Still she did not admit to anything beyond her happiness at our presence — how lovely it was we could have dinner together because surgery was delayed, and how convenient it was that there'd be pizza left over for us to take back to the hotel for tomorrow.

We all ate less than usual that evening, my mother especially so. And even though we had talked about doing something together afterwards — stopping at a favorite store in the same area and then taking the short drive to Middle Cove Beach so Kenneth and I could feel the rocks beneath our feet and breathe the rich salt air — we didn't do any of that with her. My mother explained she was tired after the exertions of the day, as of course she would be. But as we drove back to 37 Penetanguishene and dropped her off, I knew exertions were only a small part of the reason.

The sky was crystal clear blue, no clouds in sight, when Kenneth and I drove in silence without her to Middle Cove. Between 6:05 and 6:07 p.m. we captured images on my camera — rocks and ocean, and a classic seagull image set against the backdrop of blue. We didn't stay long, no more than ten minutes in total, but it was enough to ground us. Then we returned to the hotel where we unpacked the supplies we'd picked up at the grocery, and Kenneth connected his laptop to the TV so the DVD of a Corrs concert we'd brought along could be played.

On Thursday morning, after our breakfast of grocery store muffins and bananas, and after I'd arranged to change the date of our flights back to Ontario, Kenneth stayed in the room to write and edit, and spend time drinking in the view. He took photos from the window of the mist covering Signal Hill, and of the cargo ships making port to unload their containers. I went to the house to pick up my mother for one of our Saturday-like shopping trips.

There are two particularly strong impressions from that day. The first was the slowness with which my mother moved. A night's sleep had in no way eased the tiredness or reversed the frailness of the evening before. She had dressed stylishly as she always did, her hair was done, her make-up applied, and perhaps people who did not know her well would see no difference in how she carried herself. But it was glaringly obvious to me that her movements were incredibly studied and her pace so very slow.

The second was that she had absolutely no interest in looking at anything for herself. She'd always bought for others before herself — that was not unusual. Indeed, I distinctly remember asking her, when I was quite young, why she never bought anything for herself when we went shopping… and her just smiling and saying she didn't need anything. It wasn't until I was older that she explained she could only afford to buy for the children.

On this particular day she didn't say she had everything she needed for whatever time was left to her, but I knew that's what she was thinking. Instead she wanted to buy gifts for me, for Kenneth, for Peter. This also was not unusual. My mother regularly gave people gifts on days other than birthdays, anniversaries, Christmas — though of course there were presents at those times as well. She called these unexpected presents 'happy day gifts', intended to make your day happier and remind you how much you meant to someone.

She bought me two jackets that day... a reversible black fall jacket with a stand-up collar that I've worn only a few times but always remains in my closet, and a casual red windbreaker that I could wear when Kenneth and I visited Cape Spear. For Kenneth there were dry-fit golf shirts, for Peter some neckties.

I did convince her to buy deep brown lounging pajamas for herself, forcing myself to ignore the feeling that she was really only buying the outfit to humor me. They were distinctive, and the top had a collar that could stand up. My mother, you see, loved collars that could stand up. Hers always did. She also loved dark brown — it had been her signature all through my childhood before she made the switch to black after I'd begun wearing that color in my late teens. The pajamas would be appropriate for the hospital, we agreed, after the surgery when she was ready for visitors. And for home as well.

It is a distinctly disconcerting feeling to shop with someone who believes they have everything they need for the remaining short term of their lives. Someone who maintains the pretense that everything will be fine, but whose actions convey the opposite message. Someone who buys something for herself just to humor you.

I had expected a morning of shopping followed by lunch that day, but we made it to only two stores before I brought her home. She did not have the energy for more; indeed, that much activity had already been too great a drain. I stayed for a short visit, admiring the new living room furniture she'd wanted for so long and finally bought a couple of months earlier, then eased out the door.

She'd never admit that she wanted me to leave, but that is what I felt, because when the door closed and she was alone, she would be free to feel whatever it was she felt, act however she needed to act. She didn't have to put on a strong or calm facade for her daughter or grandson. If she was in pain, and clearly she was, she didn't have to try to hide it. If she needed to stop and rest as she walked from the kitchen to the bedroom, which clearly she did, she could do so.

With no one there to see, no one there who needed to be reassured that everything would be fine, she could simply be. There wasn't much I could give her, but I could give her that.

What strength my mother had. What amazing, incomparable determination.

And pride.

Day 8
Friday, May 12

I am reminded, as I relive the experiences of my mother's last weeks, that as outgoing and talkative as she was — she could talk for hours, to anyone, and no matter the circumstances, always found the right thing to say — she was also intensely private, and rarely asked for help or support. Adored by many, inside the family and out, at home and at work, she was the person everyone turned to when they needed help, and she offered all she could give of herself.

When I was little, she'd be called at all hours of the day or night when someone in the neighborhood was sick, or had fallen, or cut themselves. There'd be a knock at the door and someone would ask: *Is your mother at home? Can you ask her to come? We need her.* And she would go, spending much of her limited free time cleaning wounds, taking temperatures, sending people off to hospital when necessary. The Penetanguishene nurse.

When there were illnesses in our own family — on her side or my Dad's — she would spend all night at the hospital by someone's bedside, then go to work in that same hospital when morning arrived. She could somehow last for days on little or no sleep. It wasn't until I was a teenager that I began to realize the toll this took on her, but she couldn't have acted any differently — this was who she was.

The years she spent caring for my father as he battled Alzheimer's were perhaps the longest-running example of both how much she would give, and how little help she would accept, despite the cost to herself. I'd lived that experience with her, and it had taught me many things, one of which was how to judge what assistance she might be willing to accept, and when.

By the third day of our visit to St. John's, I had a much better sense of how little energy she had and the limits of what she was able to do. There would be no more shopping trips, and no physically taxing outings… On this day, day 8 since her diagnosis, we would simply have a quiet lunch and talk.

The restaurant we chose was relatively new, with a

simple menu that specialized in chicken and rib dishes, with excellent fries and desserts. It was rare that my mother could go anywhere in St. John's without seeing someone she knew, and this day was no different: a former student of hers, who had later become a colleague in the School of Nursing at St. Clare's Mercy Hospital, spotted us at our table just after we were seated. My mother's answer to the inevitable 'how are you?' question was by now well-rehearsed, though this did not soften its impact on Bernadette, who was going through many challenges of her own. The two women parted with a hug, and the promise to extend many prayers for the challenges they'd both face in the days to come.

When we were alone again, my mother asked if I'd mind if she ordered a glass of wine. She knew that I rarely drank alcohol — with the exception of the first weeks of my convalescence after knee surgery, when my dad would pour his 14-year-old daughter a capful of brandy to help ease her shaking and settle her stomach so she could try to eat something before physiotherapy — I'd never turned to alcohol for assistance in coping with anything.

But her question struck me as almost absurd: of course I wouldn't mind. I remember thinking that she could drink the whole bottle if it would ease the shaking of her hands just a little, and soften the lines of pain on her face.

We ordered our lunch, and began to talk about nothing of consequence. I had intended that this outing be light, the conversation about regular things — a normal lunch during an anything-but-normal time — and much of it was. However, my mother had something significant she needed to discuss with me.

Her words, as I remember them:

I know you don't want to talk about this, and maybe you won't have to worry about it for a long time, but I have to tell you something. I want to be buried in my nurse's uniform. And my hat, I want that with me but not on my head. It should be near the top of the casket and off to the side. But the uniform I prefer has short sleeves, and my arms are so thin now. I don't know what to do about that. They'll look so thin. And I'm afraid with everything being white, I'll look too pale as well. There'll be no color whatsoever. And I don't know what to do about that.

I know these conversations are necessary, and I am my mother's daughter, so while inside my mind I screamed for her to stop talking about her final outfit — for the clock to turn back and her cancer to magically go away — I simply looked at her. Because as much as it broke my heart to be even thinking about this, I knew I had the perfect answer. I knew this was one problem I could actually solve.

You should wear your nurse's cape, I told her.

The red-lined, navy blue cape would cover her arms, and she had always looked so beautiful in it. In fact, for me, the cape with the white uniform, and the white hat with black band, was the attire that best captured the essence of my mother — her warmth, her caring, her class, her style, her pride, and her strength.

The dilemma was solved, and she smiled with relief as the load was lifted from her shoulders. I have no idea what kind of expression I wore in that moment, or what kind of expression I wore later, when we returned to the house and she took me to my bedroom — with its white walls, red shag carpet, red bookshelves, desk, and *Vogue* graphic mirrors on the wall. She needed to show me where everything — uniform, slip, and undergarments — were hung inside plastic, waiting for the day when I would need to access them. The box on the shelf held her stockings and perfectly polished shoes. And there was space beside the uniform where she would hang the cape.

I can see it as clearly now as if I was standing there still; the closet that had once been packed with my clothes and shoes, where we would hide with my young cousins when it was time for their visits to end so we could delay their departure… totally empty except for the garments my mother wished to wear to her grave.

Clothes that perhaps we would not need for many years to come.

Day 9
Saturday, May 13

My mother stayed at home for the entirety of Saturday, May 13th. It was another beautiful day — the weather was uncommonly good in St. John's for that time of year — but the week had been immensely draining for her.

For Kenneth and I there was a Mother's Day present to find, and a quick visit with my best friend since seventh grade, Ann Marie Reid. Her daughter's high school graduation was that night — a formal dinner and dance in the same hotel where we were staying, and my friend Hayes (her maiden name and my name for her to this day) wanted us to come see 'Miss Amy' in a dress that was the color of sunshine. We tried to convince my mother to come with us as well, but she declined, standing in the kitchen doorway and waving us away. She was happy to stay at home, she told us, and we didn't insist that she do otherwise. How could we?

The visit with Hayes was relatively short. The afternoon and evening would be busy for their family, and Kenneth and I had a mission to complete. I had bought a Mother's Day card back in Ontario before I knew Mom was ill, but in the turmoil of getting ready, I had forgotten to bring it with me. Her gift had already been sent and received — a new set of luggage for her trip to Kenneth's graduation in June, ordered and delivered directly from the store. Locating her black suitcase among all the other black suitcases on the luggage carousel had always been something of a frustration; on this trip she would have handsome gray plaid bags that would be easy to spot, and a fashion statement as well.

But items delivered in advance of Mother's Day when we were thousands of miles apart in support of a trip that might not happen were not sufficient gifts under the new circumstances, so finding something else — even something small — was important.

It actually took less time than I anticipated to discover *A Mother's Daily Prayer Book*, by Elaine Creaseman, June Eaton, Margaret Anne Huffman, and Marie D. Jones. The cover had a beautiful pink rose, and each spread had a prayer and a verse or quote, illustrated by a flower or two. I'd been searching in vain for stargazer lilies since we had arrived in St. John's — hoping for a sign from my father that everything would somehow be fine — and I remember even now how Kenneth and I paused and looked at each other as we opened the book to the date of her diagnosis, then the date of her surgery. But there were no stargazers on either day. Instead we found that flower on May 15th, one day before her surgery.

Kenneth dubbed May 15th stargazer lily day, and we quietly contemplated what message my father was sending. We also found a card which, I didn't realize until I returned to Waterloo some time later, was the exact one I'd purchased and forgotten to bring. Finally, there was a second card — a stargazer lily on the cover and blank inside, so I could write a message to her.

I don't remember what I wrote in that card, and I can no longer find it. Perhaps one day it will appear again, perhaps it won't. I do have the book. It normally has a place on one of the sets of shelves in my home but as I write this it is beside my keyboard, open to May 15th, and to the Fran Caffey Sandin quote that spoke volumes to me at the time: "I have felt assured that I do not have to fear the future because God is already there."

Yes Dad, I thought, *I know what you are telling me. With this lily, this quote, and the card that is blank inside. I should not be so certain of the outcome of the days to come. I do not want to be so certain. I want to be surprised and amazed and able to tell a different story. I want to believe there will be another miracle. And so I shall... or at least I shall try to...*

But mostly I will try not to fear the future.

Day 10
Sunday, May 14

At 6:03 p.m. Newfoundland time on Sunday, May 14th, 2006, Kenneth and I were atop Signal Hill with dozens of other visitors and locals who had come to watch the breathtaking image of the fog rolling in after what had been a beautiful sunny afternoon. It's a view you never grow tired of, no matter how many times you see it, and if you've lived away for a decade (as we had by then) it's an experience you treasure even more.

I know the exact hour and minute because of the time stamp on the first digital photo we took there. Then, in the sixty seconds between 6:04 and 6:05, I took three photos of Kenneth that remain among my favorites. At 6:08 he took one of me in a black turtleneck, the black poncho I'd sewn the weekend before, and dark glasses, looking out over the expansive ocean. Both of us were getting lost in the sight of the fog, both of us were letting the brisk ocean air, the wind, and the purity of the place, soothe us. I didn't recognize it at the time, but later I would come to realize that everything we experienced on the trip was somehow captured in those photos, even though much of it was still yet to occur.

We had asked my mother to come with us to Signal Hill, but of course she said no. The part of the day that was significant for her — the part she'd requested, and left the house for — was already behind us. She was again completely exhausted.

We had spent the afternoon at my brother's house — mother, son, daughter, grandchildren and dogs. My brother Rik, a musician who'd been living away from Newfoundland since before our father died, had moved back to St. John's a few years prior. He lived with his wife (who was traveling at the time), two daughters, and their dogs, in a beautiful, upper class, period home in the downtown area. It was the type of home my mother admired, even if she would not have chosen it for herself. Kenneth and I had not yet seen him on this trip.

The afternoon passed as these afternoons do — what's happening on the surface masking the story that rests just beneath.

Rik's youngest daughter, Rose, and their two dogs were determined to entertain. There were tours of bedrooms, playrooms, and studios, and detailed explanations of special toys. Rik spoke of plans to someday purchase the adjoining home from the musician who owned it, and then knock out the wall in between.

We watched my mother watching the dogs, as she sat wrapped in a dark green fleece sweater on the couch. We took photos... our last captured images of her. As much as I treasure them they are heartbreaking too, because it's impossible to miss the pain and the intensity in her eyes, and the lines etched more deeply in her face, which had grown too thin.

Rik ordered Chinese takeout. There were jokes about the chicken balls with their sweet and sour sauce not being real Chinese food. There may have been dessert.

The meal complete, we drove a tired mother home, after a brief stop at a pharmacy to pick up something she would need the following day. She did not want to have to go out again on Monday.

Then Kenneth and I went to Signal Hill, because the fog was rolling in despite the sun that was, in that moment, shining.

Day 11
Monday, May 15

May in Newfoundland is not normally shirt-sleeve weather, especially at Cape Spear, the most easterly point of North America. That particular location can be bitterly cold in the middle of summer, when just a few miles away the sun is shining brightly and the temperatures are comfortably warm or even hot. But Newfoundland is more than capable of surprising you with exactly the kind of day you need exactly when you need it.

We woke early on Monday, ate breakfast in our room, layered in warm clothes meant for short hikes over uneven ground, and for sitting on rocks atop hills. Despite my obsession with packing all the right clothes, I had failed to include a warm, causal jacket, though I forgive myself that omission. I had not expected such an outing, and it was really only the delayed surgery that afforded us the opportunity to visit this favorite spot. I was therefore wearing the red jacket that had been one of my 'happy day gifts' from the abbreviated shopping trip the day after we'd arrived.

We had asked my mother to come with us before we dropped her home on Sunday night, but she had of course refused. Again, she did not want to leave her house on Monday.

That morning, Kenneth and I took turns sitting on the first bench you encounter on Cape Spear's cliff-side path, each of us staring out over the North Atlantic while the other took photos. The water was the deep blue that marks the ice-cold waves… the rocks their dark gray and brown. Both land and sea were incredibly beautiful and incredibly dangerous for any unwary person who ignored the warning signs. It was chilly enough at first to keep our jackets on, but by the time we crossed the rocky terrain up to the lighthouse, stopping to lean against the fence that needed a new coat of white paint, our jackets were tied around our waists.

There is nothing to do on these cliffs besides stand or sit or walk. You take in all that is underfoot, all that lies in front of you, all that lies behind. Cape Spear is a place both for thinking, and for not thinking. It is a place to simply be. I don't recall seeing another soul that morning, though that could be faulty memory. The sun warmed us, the breeze calmed us, and the rocks we stood upon gave us strength.

We left after a time, and drove around to Fort Amherst, the harbor-protecting fortress that we had seen countless times from the elevated vantage point on Signal Hill, but had never visited. It looked different close up, at eye level — more worn. But the coastline... what a view that offered. We stood, breathed the sea air, and took more pictures. By the time the morning was almost done we had what we needed. Wind-blown hair, lungs filled with salt air, and the strength of the rock to carry us through the days ahead.

Life intruded as soon as we found ourselves back in the city and cell phone range. A call from my office in Ontario — an HR issue to resolve. I found a spot to pull off the road to talk, part of me wondering at the absurdity of dealing with such things at this particular time. Then I dropped Kenneth back at the hotel before driving to my mother's house. She wasn't alone; an old friend had come to see her... someone she had worked with years ago. The name I knew, though I have forgotten it now;

the person I had only met once or twice before. I sat and listened, answered questions, remained silent during the observations about how much I had aged since the last time she'd seen me, when I was in university.

I stayed the afternoon, but before I left my mother insisted on showing me again the nurse's uniform hanging in what had been my closet, all the required pieces of clothing — now including the navy blue cape — organized neatly under the clear plastic coverings. The box with shoes and stockings, and the RN's cap, with its proud black band, sitting in its own plastic wrap, on the shelf.

Monday night, while my mother packed her hospital bags and talked to her sisters and friends on the phone, Kenneth and I worked in our hotel room. Perhaps we should have been with her at the house, but we weren't and I do not believe she wanted us there. She needed to sit in the chair she always occupied for evening telephone conversations, and talk as she always did with the people to whom she meant so much.

And I needed to be working with my son, so that in the morning, she and I both would be ready for the journey to the operating room.

Day 12

Tuesday, May 16

My wake-up call came around 5:00 a.m.; my mother's pick-up time was 6:30.

She was already waiting at the back door when I pulled into the driveway. She stood there, small suitcase by her feet and purse over her shoulder, with all the doors and windows closed behind her except the final one — a glass storm door — that she stepped through as I stopped the car and got out.

I wouldn't get to see her one last time in the kitchen, or in her chair in the living room, or putting the final touches on her make-up in her bedroom. If there were goodbyes for her to say, she had already said them. If there were images for me to preserve, they would have to exist already in my memories.

My mother had spent the majority of her life in hospitals, but it only occurs to me now, years after that particular day, that I had not previously taken her to hospital for some illness of her own. Maybe a medical appointment or two over the years, but she had infrequently been a patient in my presence.

We checked her in and I sat with her in the long rectangular room where those destined for surgery wait for their name to be called. In my memory the walls are cold and green, and the room harsh and metal. I don't think it was actually like that, but it's how I perceived this place.

My mother had completed her nursing training at this same hospital — St. Clare's Mercy Hospital. After she'd been forced to stop working in Emergency (the area she loved best) because of the gastric hemorrhage she suffered when I was five-years-old, she'd become a nursing instructor, and everywhere in the building were nurses who at one point had been her students. The majority of them had called her 'Mom'; the care she showed them earned her that honor, and it is no exaggeration to say she was widely adored.

Because of this, I knew without a doubt that she would have the best possible care — these former students would repay her kindnesses and prove that they had learned well from her.

My dearest friend Hayes, who we'd visited briefly on Saturday, now worked in the Operating Room and was on duty that day. She came to see us while we waited. She wouldn't be in my mother's surgery, but would check on her as often as she could and provide me with updates whenever possible. For me, she was a lifeline.

When they came to wheel my mother away, we were waiting at the farthest end of the room from the doors through which patients exited, and I watched from there until she was out of sight. Then I clutched her bags and mine, walked to another, smaller rectangular waiting room, and sat in one of the wooden-armed, leather chairs. Eventually I pulled out pages I had brought with me to edit. They were a familiar weight on my lap, a familiar job to occupy some of my thoughts. The mechanical pencil in my hand was a comfort.

My brother Rik stopped by after he dropped his daughters at school. I have always been quieter than either of my brothers, so Rik contributed more to our conversation than I did. This was not unusual; every so often my mother used to remind me of an image she held of me in her mind. I was still young enough to be in a playpen, and on this particular day, I was wearing little red plaid pants and a white sweater. As was apparently my habit, I was observing what was going on with great intent, but saying nothing. My mother thought: *Poor little thing, how's she ever going to get on in the world if she never says a word?*

We used to laugh about that later, once I'd grown. I'd tell her: *Of course I didn't talk much. Between you, Steve, Rik and all our visitors, how was I supposed to get a word in edgewise?* The reality, though, was that I was more like my father in that regard. We tend towards quiet — listen more than we talk.

My Aunt Sheila came from her home in Ferryland, the historic outport on the Southern Shore where the fourteen Morry children in my mother's family had grown up, and joined us in the waiting room early in the day.

Sheila, the youngest of the seven sisters, is strength and beauty and laughter. She's a wildly entertaining storyteller, and blessed with what we used to call the 'Morry gift of gab.' She'd lived in Labrador for much of my life so I'd only met her briefly when she came to St. John's for visits, and didn't really have any chance to get to know her until the last weeks of my father's life. She'd come to visit my mother when she happened to be in town. She stayed for many days when she realized what was happening, saving us then with her stories and her laughter. She stayed with me that day too, so I would not be alone — saving me again with her stories and her laughter and her strength.

Time moves all too slowly in these waiting rooms, and moves slower still once the hands of the clock move past the time you were told you could expect the surgery to be over. Sometime in the early afternoon, Hayes came to tell us that my mother was in the recovery room, but they needed to keep her there longer. Something about difficulties they hadn't anticipated.

The next time she came it was to let us know my mother was being moved to the Intensive Care Unit, instead of a regular room as had been the original plan, and would have been the norm. The exact reason is blurry now, but there had been complications, and they needed to monitor her.

I still had my mother's small suitcase and purse with me, but since she wouldn't need them that evening, Sheila and I took them to the car before she left to head home. Sheila, I recall, wouldn't let me carry anything, because I'd had surgery just a few weeks before.

The rest of the day was spent waiting. Checking in with Kenneth and Peter back at home in Ontario. With Steve in BC. And waiting. Waiting outside the ICU for the doctor to come and tell me what had happened, what he had found, what to expect. Waiting for Hayes because she was my link to the nurses inside ICU.

Waiting for a doctor who didn't come. Waiting for Hayes, who always did. Waiting for news.

At some point I got a muffin from the hospital cafeteria — I hadn't eaten all day and needed to. Finally, sometime after 8 p.m., when I learned the doctor had, in fact, left the hospital and wouldn't be coming to see me, I departed too. On shaky legs and an empty stomach.

The image of my mother being wheeled away in her chair etched firmly in my mind.

Day 13
Wednesday, May 17

My memories of May 17th are divided into three distinct parts: a morning visit to Intensive Care so a grandson could see his grandmother; a surreal afternoon settling my mother into a private room on the sixth floor of St. Clare's Mercy Hospital; and an evening defined by a piece of carrot cake.

I'll start with the third: the carrot cake, and the kindness it reflected — a kindness that still reaches deep inside, and fills my eyes with tears. The definition, for me, of friendship.

I'd eaten virtually nothing for two days — hadn't wanted to. But at some point in the late afternoon I started to feel some semblance of appetite return and I began wishing for carrot cake. I said as much to Hayes when she somehow managed another visit to my mother's room. *The only thing I really want is a piece of carrot cake,* I told her.

I shouldn't have been surprised when the phone rang about forty-five minutes after I got back to the hotel room that evening. I shouldn't have been surprised that it was Hayes. She was downstairs, and needed the room number. She'd gone home after her long shift (a shift interrupted by trips to check on my mother and me) and had gotten her husband Bruce (Saint Bruce, she rightfully calls him) to drive her back into town from their home outside the city so she could buy carrot cake and bring it to my downtown hotel. The process must have added at least an hour and a half to her already long day.

I cried after the door closed behind her, standing there with the cake in my hands as she headed home for the second time that evening, to make dinner for her family. Or, I should say, for *the rest* of her family.

This was Newfoundland. And this was Hayes, the best friend anyone could ever ask for.

• • •

Rewind about six or seven hours. My mother had been released from ICU, and she would need her bags and everything in them — or so I thought. While the nurses settled her into her bed, I retrieved the bags from the car, my step lighter than it had been the previous day.

When I saw her for the first time after the surgery, her frailty was still a surprise, and the oxygen tube was disturbing. I hung her clothes in the room's closet — she wouldn't be able to wear any of them at that point, but maybe tomorrow. Her prayer-a-day book and stargazer lily card found a place on a small shelf inset into the wall. She couldn't really see them from her vantage point, but they were there for her anyway. Or maybe for the visitors.

Nurses, in my mother's day, wore outfits like the one she wanted to be buried in — spotless white uniforms, hats with the black band that marked their status as RNs, white stockings and shoes that were meticulously cared for. The nurses who tended her after her surgery wore the garments of the mid-2000s: smocks with pants and sneaker-like shoes — all colors, nothing uniform-like about them. She cooperated with her caregivers, was polite, but when they left the room she would comment sadly about their shoes and lack of uniforms.

Visitors, expecting a much more robust Mary, began flooding in. Most stayed just a short time when they realized rest was what she most needed. Some stayed a long time, sitting quietly in case she needed anything. We were relieved, because she was out of ICU and surely that meant she was improving.

• • •

Rewind further, back to the late morning. At that point we didn't know how long my mother would be in Intensive Care, but Kenneth and I were scheduled to return to Ontario the following day, so this would likely be the best opportunity for him to see her before he left. And seeing her was necessary, in case she wasn't able to come for his graduation in June after all.

I suspect if we'd been able to ask, my mother would have told us she didn't want Kenneth to visit her, especially in ICU. The image of her in bed, with oxygen tubes and surrounded by all manner of monitoring devices, is not the picture she would want to leave her grandson. She would fear, I think, that this sort of mental image would override all the others in his memory.

But it was a visit that needed to happen, which is something she would have also understood.

Kenneth found the hospital was quite different than the gleaming marvels of future technology he included in his novels at the time. In the futures he imagined, the

ICU's sense of weariness is replaced by hope and energy — the knowledge that any malady might be overcome by the wisdom of doctors like Elandra Caine. This ICU was different. The carefully-erected barrier (he calls it an 'airlock') that separated it from the rest of the hospital. The hand sanitizer stations. The monitoring devices, the nearby nurses, and the oxygen... these are what he remembers.

He doesn't remember how long we stood by the bed — not long, I suspect — or what we said — just a little, if anything. He was aware that this might be the last time he saw his grandmother, and he knew her fate was out of his hands.

We were three generations there in the ICU — in a place none of us wanted to be.

Day 14
Thursday, May 18

Fog, in Newfoundland, has a particular character. There have been times in my life when it has felt intentional, almost sentient — as if it has come when it is needed, to wrap a soft blanket around me, protect me while I worked inside myself to find a way through some harsh reality.

On Thursday, May 18th, fog infused everything... a light fog at first, then a thicker, denser, heavier fog that caused the world to pause.

Kenneth and I were scheduled to fly out mid-afternoon. Steve was coming in the evening, so I had no worries that my mother would lack for the company and care she needed. Indeed, as a doctor he would know what questions to ask and what signs or symptoms to look for — things I didn't know. And his presence would bring her happiness, if anything could.

We packed early in the morning, a light fog blurring the view of Signal Hill from our window. Then I visited my mother in the hospital, a final visit before my flight. When I had left the night before, the nurses had expected she would be improved in the morning, so my step was again a bit light when I walked down the hall to her room.

But she was not improved, really. Not worse, but not better. Still weak, and tired, and the oxygen was still required. They were monitoring some fluid build-up in one of her lungs, which years prior had been damaged by tuberculosis. This was not abnormal, they told me — it was expected to clear.

And Steve would be there in less than twelve hours.

By the time we reached the airport, the fog had gotten thicker. We sat at our departure gate, Kenneth and I, wondering if the flight would actually be able to leave. Wondering if the fog was telling us that we should be staying — that to leave now was to somehow desert my mother when she needed us most. We talked about that — should we go back through security and ask to reschedule the flight?

But I knew, in the place I've learned to never question, that I was supposed to at least try to get Kenneth home that day, and I'm as certain about that now as I was then. I also knew I had to get home as well — had to escape St. John's that day, if it was at all possible, even if it meant I had to come back.

So we sat and waited, positioned in front of a wall of windows through which only the faintest outline of a plane was visible beneath the heavy shroud of fog. Waited through the first flight delay, then the second. Waited until late in the afternoon when the fog slipped back beyond the horizon and told us it was time to leave.

For now.

Day 15
Friday, May 19

I went to my office on Friday, May 19th. I needed normality. I needed to think about something that wasn't related to illness, and didn't involve hospitals. Between my surgery and my mother's, I'd been away from my desk for weeks. I needed, on so many levels, to be there.

On my way home from work, I stopped at a store that I wandered through some days for no other purpose than to decompress. I was still there when Steve called me, to give me the latest update and tell me he needed me to come back to Newfoundland.

Steve and I had talked frequently throughout the day. My mother's condition had not improved or even stabilized in the twenty-four hours since Kenneth and I had boarded the plane in St. John's. Indeed, the fluid build-up in her lungs had gotten worse throughout the night and was an escalating concern, as was her dependence on oxygen and her decreasing strength and lucidity. Pneumonia, they had decided. Apparently, the tuberculosis-damaged lung was much weaker than anyone in the family would ever have realized.

As I stood in an aisle by the picture frames and listened to Steve's voice, I learned she required more constant monitoring and care than was available in her regular room. With his encouragement, they were returning her to the ICU.

While I was relieved to know that she would be receiving the attention she needed, I was entirely aware of what the need for constant monitoring and care meant. I was also beginning to realize, just as we all were, that the tuberculosis she had survived as a young woman had been far more damaging than any of us had realized. Whether she was aware of that, whether she concealed that truth for her entire life, I will never know. Whether we should have predicted the danger ourselves, I cannot say. Perhaps we can be forgiven for never having guessed that my active, vibrant mother had lived the majority of her life on anything less than two lungs with full capacity.

But even had we known she'd been left with a lung ill-equipped to deal with the stress it was now enduring, there would have been no choice but to proceed with the surgery.

Steve believed that if the deterioration in her current condition continued, it would proceed rapidly, so we had very little time. As a family, we needed to decide what our mother had meant when she'd told Rik she never wanted to be on life support.

I had boarded a plane just over twenty-four hours earlier... brought Kenneth home... hugged and commiserated with cancer-fighting Atlas... held Peter through the night... gone to my office and done normal things for about eight hours... then stopped at a favorite store on the way home to look at picture frames and journals and housewares.

One regular day of respite, to partially restore the balance of my life... but now I headed home to update Peter and Kenneth, call my boss, book another flight, and pack another suitcase.

A suitcase filled with what-if clothes.

Day 16
Saturday, May 20

Now everything speeds up; at the same time it slows down.

Hayes picked me up at the airport mid-afternoon on Saturday. I almost had more luggage than her blue hatchback could accommodate — uncertain as I was of the length of my trip and the circumstances I would face, my packing had been, for want of a better word, thorough.

We stopped quickly at my mother's house so I could drop off my suitcase and garment bag — leave them unopened in my childhood bedroom. Then it was on to the hospital where we would have the first of too few family conferences about my mother's treatment options.

When I'd boarded the plane in the morning, I knew my mother's condition was continuing to deteriorate. Rik had said she'd told him that she didn't want to be kept alive on machines. *No life support,* her words had been. I can imagine her saying them. I can hear the tone she would have used and picture the look on her face as easily as if I had been present to witness the instructions.

But did that mean she wouldn't have wanted assistance while receiving treatment that could help with the pneumonia and give her time to heal? What exactly did 'life support' mean and at what point did the 'no life support' directive kick in? Could she possibly want us to just let her go, without trying to save her?

So many families are forced to ask themselves these questions. I wish that there were easier answers, but there are not.

I can't recall who else was there that day when Hayes and I reached the hospital. I remember only my two brothers, Hayes — who we asked to please stay, she was family too — and the female doctor who came to speak with us.

You never want to hear the words you inevitably hear in these rooms with doctors who are so practiced in their deliveries. The words trying to prepare you for things that make no sense and outcomes that can't possible be real. Outcomes they would know were wrong if only they knew your mother. The same mother who had already told her daughter exactly what clothes she wanted to be buried in.

The doctor's concern was clinical and legitimate: what if we managed to deal with the immediate danger? What if antibiotics helped address the pneumonia? There was still the cancer to deal with. The possibility of chemo seemed remote at best; based on my mother's age and her general physical condition, she likely wouldn't survive it. So why prolong the inevitable? Our mother wasn't a young woman.

I thought: *How can you think of our mother as old? You don't know her. You don't know how much she has done, how much she still has to do, how vibrant she has always been, the struggles she has overcome in her lifetime, the battles she has won, the difference she has made in this very hospital, the lives she has helped save... You don't know her. And if there's any chance at all that she can beat the odds, shouldn't we at least give her the chance? How can we sit in this room and give up on someone who never gave up on anyone else?*

We didn't have to make the decision right then, at least. Things weren't critical that afternoon. But they were heading in that direction, and when they reached a certain point, the choice before us would be whether to intubate — to ease the strain on her lungs so that the antibiotics would have time to work. We had hours, maybe a whole day, before the decision would need to be made.

That afternoon I made the first of many trips into the surreal world of the ICU. Through the outer, then inner doors — Kenneth's 'airlock' — then a right turn to take me to my mother's bed. She recognized me, knew I had come to visit, but she wasn't surprised to see me. I don't think she realized that I had flown home two days before, and was now back again, less than forty-eight hours later.

We spoke, but not about anything of significance. Silently, I learned to understand the readings on the monitor over her bed, so I would know what to look for in the vigil that would follow.

When we eventually left the hospital that evening, Steve, Hayes, and I went to a downtown restaurant for dinner. Of all the things I could remember, I remember the underground parking. I don't remember the food. I don't remember the conversation.

Then Steve and I went back to the house we had

grown up in — me to my old bedroom, him to the one right beside it that he'd shared with Rik before moving to his own room in the basement. The furniture in his room was different than it had been — it was furniture we had given her when we first left Newfoundland. The furniture in my room was the same, a minor detail that was almost a metaphor for the very moment in time we found ourselves trapped within.

He slept — he felt a distinct comfort in being home.

I didn't — I couldn't even get under the covers of the tiny twin bed that had been my refuge for years. The small bedside lamp stayed on all night. The house, without either my mother or my father, was haunted by grief, beset by hollow horror.

My room, with my mother's casket clothes hanging in the closet, was a place I couldn't bear to be.

Day 17
Sunday, May 21

May 20th, 2006 was the last night I would ever spend in my parents' home, though I don't think I realized that when I called the hotel on Sunday morning.

If there was guilt at running away — for that's what it felt like I was doing — it was sufficiently overshadowed by my acceptance that I was incapable of staying.

The hotel welcomed me back, gave me a room with a view of St. John's Harbour and Signal Hill. When I could eat, a hot turkey sandwich with dressing, fries and gravy that has yet to be matched, was delivered on a tray to my room. I was also with family, literally: Aunt Sheila's daughter Nikki worked at the front desk, and one of the gifts of this time was the small chance it afforded us to get to know one another as we never had growing up. Her hugs and smiles were lifelines. Her friends and colleagues made this place a sanctuary.

This was not just for me; the hospitality and caring of Newfoundlanders is legendary. I believe it's founded in their innate generosity combined with an understanding of loss that's etched into their souls as deeply as the lines carved into the island's many cliffs.

The hotel was very near the hospital — they were, respectively, at the bottom and top of one of the famously steep hills of downtown St. John's. I simply needed to make a right turn out of the hotel's underground lot, head up that twisty hill and through one set of lights, then turn left onto the small lane outside the hospital's main entrance, park, and take an elevator to the fifth floor to be near my mother.

The waiting area was outside the outer doors to ICU, tucked at the end of a hall for some privacy, and it was mostly full that afternoon. People were arriving now as news spread, many driving hours to reach the hospital. Even though they could see my mother for only a few brief minutes, they didn't just visit her bedside and leave. They waited with us — aunts and uncles and cousins and friends, many of whom I had not seen in years, and Steve had not seen even longer.

We intubated that evening after another doctor-family conference. We had decided that an interim measure designed to ease the stress on my mother's system so that she had a chance to rally wasn't life support, per se. Every breath had been taking more and more effort, and none of them were giving her sufficient oxygen. Any chance that the antibiotics could work was being undermined by that struggle, and the related impact on kidneys and other systems was growing critical.

She knew and understood the plan: intubate, ease the pressure on her system, and give the drugs a chance to do their job. For how long, we didn't know. What the ultimate result would be, we didn't know. But at least we had hope.

When Mary Louise Barron looked up at me from her bed that day and said *remember, I will be with you always,* I should have realized that she didn't believe she would wake up. But it wasn't until later that it truly registered, and I came to understand that this was perhaps why she hadn't argued against the assisted breathing in the first place.

As evening moved to night, the sense of relief at the ease to her struggle was welcome. Hayes and I still kept vigil in the waiting area, checking regularly for updates to make sure all was well. Talking. Popping back into the room from time to time to watch the numbers on the monitors. Settling back in the waiting area again. Talking some more. By the time I returned to the hotel that night, my mother was resting peacefully, and with the lights of the harbor twinkling outside my window, I slept.

My mother would have hated, I know, to be remembered as she appeared on those days and nights in her hospital bed. But there is no worry in that regard. Because Mom, know that even now I cannot actually picture you in that bed, still wearing a hospital robe, supported by tubes and wires and all manner of machinery. There is not a single mental image of you from that time. Instead, I picture you in the long winter-white and black plaid coat you sewed, the one you always wore with the collar up... with black slacks, black turtleneck and stylish black leather shoes. Or the moss green boiled wool coat and black hat we bought on your first trip to Waterloo. Or your blue jeans, white collared shirt, and gray sweater for cold days at Bellevue. Or your white nurse's uniform and spotless white shoes.

And always, your eyes are happy and you are smiling.

Day 18
Monday, May 22

For reasons that are painfully obvious, Intensive Care Units don't have strict visiting hours. When I left the hospital on Sunday night, the nurses suggested an 11:00 arrival on Monday morning, unless we received a call suggesting we were needed sooner.

The telephone didn't ring through the night — my mother had been peaceful, her vitals improving. Monday felt lighter for that reason. After checking in at the appointed hour and sitting with her for awhile, I resumed my post in the waiting area. At regular intervals I'd make the trip through first the outer, then the inner doors, to sit or stand by her bedside. Heavily sedated as she was, she didn't know I was there, and talking wouldn't have been possible even if she did. Intubation is not conducive to conversation. But I was there anyway, my head tilted up and my eyes locked on the main monitor as I gained comfort from the numbers, and prayed the positive trend would continue.

There are sounds in an ICU you think you'll never forget. You take them with you when you leave in the evening and you hear them in your dreams all through the night. But time has taught me that after a period they do in fact dim, their meaning begins to fade, and eventually they grow silent.

I knew every nuance that day, however. People continued to visit, popping in to stand briefly at the end or side of her bed, keeping me company when I was in the waiting area, saying their own prayers. Sheila, Laura, Ursula, Flo, Esther, Mary Rogers, Betty, Jack, Kelly — aunts, uncles, cousins, my mother's friends, and Hayes of course, whenever she could.

I don't know what I ate that day. I don't know if I managed to do any editing while I sat in the waiting area, though I did bring it with me — a black leather knapsack always filled but rarely opened. What was most important was that by the time the skies had darkened and I was leaving again, the woman in the bed with the machines and assistive technologies appeared to be rallying.

As I walk this particular lane of memories, it is hard to feel again the lightness I allowed myself to feel that night. In retrospect, I know it was really nothing more than an illusion... the sun breaking briefly through the clouds, giving us a ray of hope that the skies would clear.

Which, of course, they wouldn't.

Day 19
Tuesday, May 23

My brother Steve celebrates his birthday four days before mine each year, on May 23rd.

When we returned on Tuesday morning at the appointed hour, we weren't expecting to be told my mother had improved sufficiently that the doctor thought she should be removed from the intubator. But that was the news and recommendation that awaited us.

We sat outside while the intubation process was reversed less than forty-eight hours after it had been initiated — surprised but not unhappy that it was happening so quickly.

I was on the other side of the bed when Steve leaned in to ask my mother if she knew what day it was and to thank her for his birthday gift — for rallying. I listened when he told her that just as they'd left the hospital together after he'd been born some fifty years prior, they were going to leave the hospital together again soon. I watched when she nodded back.

There will always be a question in my mind as to whether or not my mother would have survived if she had remained intubated. Would she have been able to gain more strength, or would she have become too dependent on the assistance — gotten to the stage that it would indeed have become actual life support? Also, if she had survived the post-operative ordeal, would she have been strong enough to fight the cancer? But the questions are pointless, because questions like those have no answers.

The one thing I do know is that my mother would never have allowed herself to die on Steve's birthday. She could not have shadowed the celebration of his birth with the anniversary of her death — she adored him too much, loved him too deeply.

Once my mother was breathing again on her own, the vigil of her vital signs once more became my focus. She was hoarse when they removed the tube from her throat, and still exhausted, but more lucid and aware than she had been since my return on Saturday.

I stationed myself again in the waiting area, kept company by aunts, uncles, cousins, my mother's friends, and Hayes. I returned to her bedside at times of my choosing, or when she happened to ask for one of her children. I left the hospital only for the time required to join my brothers for the birthday dinner Rik had arranged for Steve that evening.

There are parts of that day I can hardly bear to remember, yet they remain impossible to forget. All that really mattered, as the minutes of May 23rd ticked by, was what was happening to my mother physically, mentally, and emotionally. As she told me when she and I were alone and she felt strong enough to speak, she actually hadn't expected to wake up, and couldn't believe she was going to live.

Her questions to me were incredulous: *I'm getting better? I'm going to live?*

Maybe I should have answered yes to both, but I didn't. Instead I told her only what I knew to be the truth: that her oxygen levels and all her vitals had improved much over the past couple of days... that she was stronger than she had been... that everyone hoped and prayed the positive trend would continue.

And all we could do was wait to see what the overnight hours, and the next day, would bring.

Day 20
Wednesday, May 24

Based on the pace of my mother's deterioration after the intubation was removed, I suspect the date on her obituary would indeed have been May 23rd if we hadn't given the antibiotics time to fight the post-op pneumonia.

As morning moved to afternoon on Wednesday, May 24th, the advances made on Sunday night and Monday began to steadily reverse. It was as though a large ball of snow had been pushed up a hill, with every indication being that it would reach the top and stabilize. But it didn't make it. Instead, not so near to the top, it began to slide backwards, and then began rolling back down, gaining more speed with every inch.

For Steve, this was one of the hardest things of all. His life is helping people live, but he had been powerless to help his father, and now again was powerless to help his mother.

By mid-afternoon family conferences were again being called, and Steve and Rik summoned back to the hospital to discuss alternatives. There was nothing to be gained by intubation; if it hadn't worked the first time, it would not work the second. This time, any intervention would truly be life support — something she had herself now made clear to the doctor and nurses she did not want, would not permit.

We would not re-intubate, unless she specifically and lucidly requested that we do so, which wasn't going to happen. A face mask? If she allowed it, yes, but otherwise no. Just an oxygen tube for as long as she was willing.

My mother took her fate into her own hands that afternoon, fueled by a refusal to live the kind of life she knew she would have if she survived. She would undoubtedly need oxygen on an ongoing basis. Chemotherapy, if she was strong enough to have it, would take a terrible toll. Her independence would be gone. Her dignity. Chances were she would not be able to see to her own needs; people — relatives, friends or caregivers — would have to come to the house to help her.

She could not, would not, impact the lives of her

family and friends that way. She could not, would not, live like that.   There would be no more intubation, despite her again weakening state.

It's OK Mom, we weren't going to force it on you, I thought as I again sat by her bed.

She just wanted to go home to die, she told my aunts that same day. She was so angry with us, they thought, for trying to keep her alive. It broke their hearts, and mine.

I'm sorry Mom, but we had to give you a fighting chance. I know you never expected to live — the uniform in my closet, all pressed and ready for the funeral home was a clear enough message — but there was a chance you would rally. And can't you see we never could have lived with ourselves if we'd just let you go? Can't you see we had to try?

And as for taking you home to die, you were too weak to return to Penetanguishene. But St. Clare's was in some ways as much your home... with all the years you spent there... all the nurses who called you Mom. If you couldn't be in the bed you shared with my father for more than forty years, at least you could still be surrounded by love, in a place you loved as well. A place where you took away pain, saved lives, and taught others to do the same. A place where you did your life's work.

The snowball that had been moving upwards with such hope was rolling back down the hill. It was unclear how long it would continue on this downward path, but there was no longer any doubt about its destination.

Day 21
Thursday, May 25

When we arrived at the hospital on the morning of May 25th, my mother was determined and in complete control. By this I do not mean she was physically stronger; in that regard her condition had reverted to where it would have been had we not intubated on Sunday night — grown worse in fact.

But it was as if her physical and mental capacities were inversely proportional to one another — the more she lost on the physical side, the more she seemed to gain in mental strength. This was not really a surprise to those of us who knew her best, and had witnessed her mental strength while growing up, then especially during the years of my father's illness.

She had already made her wishes known to the doctor and medical staff: she would accept no additional support on that or future days, beyond what was required to ensure she could see and speak with the people to whom she wanted to say goodbye. After that, there was to be no interference. The time had come to let her go.

We talked to her, Steve and I — asked if she knew what her instructions meant, needing to be sure of her certainty and lucidity. That confirmed, we left her bedside temporarily to make the telephone calls to people she most wanted to see. Because while it was possible she would linger, rally even, there was only a miniscule chance that she would be with us by the time the sun set.

I still have a small card I made to carry in my wallet on that second trip in May 2006 — one with the home and cell numbers for Sheila, Flo, Esther, Hayes, and others. I don't remember which calls we made directly, though there were only a few. The system, never formalized but still flawless, ensured that the moment a handful of people knew, the news would spread to all the others.

Our waiting area was moved inside the outer doors of the ICU now, to a room that had soft seats and gentle lighting. This was a place meant to offer comfort for families during the final hours. I would describe it in more detail if I could, but I can't. That's all I remember.

Soon the room was full, then overfull with people

spilling out into the hall. Aunts, uncles, cousins, and friends funneled in one or two at a time to say hello, and then goodbye. No one tried to really control the flow. There was no longer any need for rest periods.

This was the morning when I asked my mother whether there was a sign I should look for, and told my aunts that there would be one — but I would only tell them what it was after I saw it.

By midday, my mother had been moved to a private room within ICU, the place where stays were to be short-term. The few belongings that had been in the drawer of her bedside table had been transferred to an identical unit there, and the machinery was all the same. But there were walls for privacy instead of curtains, and an extra chair or two.

I moved back and forth from my mother's side to the waiting room, not surprised by all the people who had come, only by the speed with which they arrived. Even my mother's family doctor, who had so quickly arranged the appointment with the specialist just twenty-one days before, came for a lunchtime visit. She wanted to tell me personally that the results of my mother's regular mammogram had arrived that morning. On any other day the news would have been chilling: the cancer, it seems, had not been isolated in my mother's abdomen after all.

Of course it hadn't, I thought.

The sound of my mother's labored breathing was the memory that haunted me most for months after her death, but I can no longer hear the ragged, struggling sounds. Thankfully, those echoes have faded. I sat alone at the foot of her bed for brief intervals, not wanting to be there, but not wanting to be anywhere else. Moving to her side to hold her hand from time to time. Leaving when someone arrived for a private moment.

Everyone I spoke with who visited my mom that day left with a message just for them. The conversations were brief — her voice was so raspy, her breathing increasingly labored — but still she managed, during her final hours, to say the things the people who meant so much to her needed to hear.

Still she managed to find the strength to be the woman who I would always remember as my mother.

By about 3:00 p.m. the stream of visitors had ended, and I was alone again at the foot of the bed. Sometime soon after the nurse who checked on her vitals looked in my direction.

Your brothers should be here, she told me.

I didn't react at first, unable to immediately process the implications. Then I suddenly realized hours had been reduced to minutes.

I can't remember if I asked the nurse if she could go to the waiting room to get Steve and Rik, or if I went. My next clear memory is of all three siblings in the room, and the nurse asking my mother if she wanted oxygen.

Will it make it easier, my mother asked, *easier to breathe?*

Yes, it will help, the nurse responded.

No, my mother insisted. *NO. NO. NO.*

She had said her goodbyes. Her children were with her. Her husband, her parents, and so many others awaited her. She would not linger; and she would leave entirely on her own terms.

It was really only minutes then, even if it seemed longer. Steve held her hand and spoke words only she would be able to hear. Each side and the foot of the bed guarded by a son or daughter listening for the next breath, watching the numbers on the monitor fall.

Then her anguished breathing finally stopped.

You miss a last breath because you don't realize it is indeed the final one until after there are no more. Her heart still beat for a brief spell after that, but not long. And the numbers on the screen didn't all fall to zero right away. Things weren't instantaneous like you see on television. But she was gone.

Obviously and finally gone, after just twenty-one days in May.

Strong, determined, and with help from no one.

Her children standing next to her.

From the small drawer unit by her bed, I gathered the items that would need to go home, or back to the people who had brought them for her, then made sure the nurses knew what had to go with her to the morgue. I went to the outer waiting room and called home to tell Peter and Kenneth that she had died, and my office to tell my boss, Arthur. Then I sat there with Hayes and Esther, literally not knowing what to do or where to go until my best friend took me in hand, guided me out of the hospital, and accompanied me to my mother's house. We had to ensure everything was organized for the following day.

Of course, I didn't stay the night in that place. Before darkness fell I was back in the sanctuary of my hotel, with my view of the Narrows.

Peter would be on a flight the following day. The clothes I would need for the wake and funeral were already hanging in the closet of the hotel, the clothes my mother would need in my childhood bedroom. In that moment, there was nothing to do. And so I stood in the middle of the room and wept, standing until I could no longer stand, crying until there were no tears left.

Then I got up again and walked to the desk, with my mother's strength and example to sustain me, and sat at my laptop to write her obituary.

BARRON, Mary L. (nee Morry), R.N. — Passed peacefully on **Thursday, May 25, 2006** at St. Clare's Mercy Hospital, **Mary Barron**, age 77 years, after a brief battle with cancer. Predeceased by her husband Richard J. in 1994. Left with loving memories her son Steve and daughter-in-law Glenna of Anmore, BC; her son Rik and daughter-in-law Sarah and granddaughters: Mae and Rose of St. John's; her daughter Jacqui Tam and son-in-law

Peter and grandson Kenneth of Waterloo, ON. Also left to mourn brother Jack (Margaret), Bishop's Falls; sisters: Ursula Kieley, Laura Morry-Williams, Sheila Morry (Aubrey Paul) all of Ferryland; Margaret Bulko (Joe) of Maryland, USA; brothers-in-law and sisters-in-law and their families: Pat and Vonnie Barron of Alberta, Lawrence and Jo Barron of Mount Pearl, Marg Barron of Prince Edward Island, Jim and Flo Barron of St. John's, Theresa and Bill Janes, Cole Hr., NS; as well as countless nieces, nephews and numerous close friends and nursing colleagues. Resting at Carnell's Funeral Home, 329 Freshwater Road on Saturday and Sunday from 2-4 and 7-9 p.m. Mass of Christian Burial will take place on Monday, May 29, 2006 at 1:30 p.m. from St. Pius X Parish with interment to follow at Holy Sepulchre Cemetery. Flowers gratefully accepted or donations in Mary's memory may be made to the Dr. H. Bliss Murphy Cancer Care Foundation or St. Clare's Mercy Hospital. To send a message of condolence or to sign the memorial guest book, please visit *www.carnells.com.*

The level of strength and courage with which you lived your life amazed and touched everyone you knew. The strength and courage you displayed in these last weeks and in your last hour astounded even those of us who knew you so very well. You were a remarkable woman, and loving wife, mother, daughter, sister, aunt, friend and nurse. We will miss you, we will love you, and we will celebrate you forever. (Published 05/27/06)

Epilogue

On the Monday we buried my mother, her coffin was escorted into the church by an honor guard of nurses, and guided to its place in front of the altar by her son-in-law, Peter, brother Jack, three nephews, Vincent, Peter and Pat, and dear friend Mario.

As I knelt in the front-row pew after Holy Communion, Peter at my side, the nurses slowed so very slightly to touch my hand as they walked past. Of course these nurses would understand the incredible power of their gentle touches. Of course they would also know how important it was that any goodbye to my mother include them — she had organized so many such guards herself over the years, it was only fitting that she be honored in the same manner.

Our dear Penetanguishene neighbor, Nora, who'd been my piano teacher when I was little, was the organist.

My cousins Wynn-Ann, Lynn, Todd, and Nikki, and Rik's wife Sarah, all played a role in the service. The beautiful voices of cousin Margaret, Aunt Lillian's daughter, and her own daughter Anna, filled the church with *On Eagles Wings*. And as her casket left the church, it was accompanied by Rik's instrumental *Hand in Hand*.

Steve and I had chosen her casket together. It was wooden, with beautiful rose etchings. I knew instantly it was the correct one. The certainty I felt the moment I saw it didn't surprise me. Steve knew instantly as well, but was startled by the physical jolt that went through him. It was disconcerting, but powerful, and not a sensation he'd expected or previously experienced, he explained to me later. I just smiled. *That was Mom making sure you knew this was the one she wanted,* I told him.

The traditional Newfoundland wake had been held on Saturday and Sunday, the room constantly packed with people. I was usually the first person visitors had approached at the funeral home. *You have to be Jacqui,* they'd say. *You look so much like your mother did at your age.*

Many of the people who'd taken the time to come to the wake attended the funeral as well, filling the parking lot and the church. My mother had feared the church wouldn't be full — we'd talked about that at our last lunch too. I'd reassured her then, and now I imagined her looking down and being content at the sight below her.

I met many of these people again outside the church in the parking lot. Thanked them for coming. There were hugs, memories, smiles, tears, and a lingering disbelief that it would take all of us a while to shake, if we ever truly did. And goodbyes. So many of these people I would not see again for a very long time. Some I would not see ever.

We lowered my mother into her place next to my father, then returned for the post-funeral gathering to the house where I'd grown up. The place I'd fled from days before. Aunts, uncles, cousins, the dearest of friends — they were all there, with food and drink, laughter and stories, and moments when everything would just suddenly grow quiet.

When Peter and I left to head back to the hotel and pack — we were flying out the next morning — I thought I'd be back in the summer, to help empty and ready the house for sale. But I never did go back... never stepped through the back door again. Maybe I couldn't.

Maybe the truth is that I didn't need to.

My mother was no longer there, and never would be again.

But her courage and her strength, her determination and her dedication, her style and her class, and all the lessons she had taught me, these would be with me always.

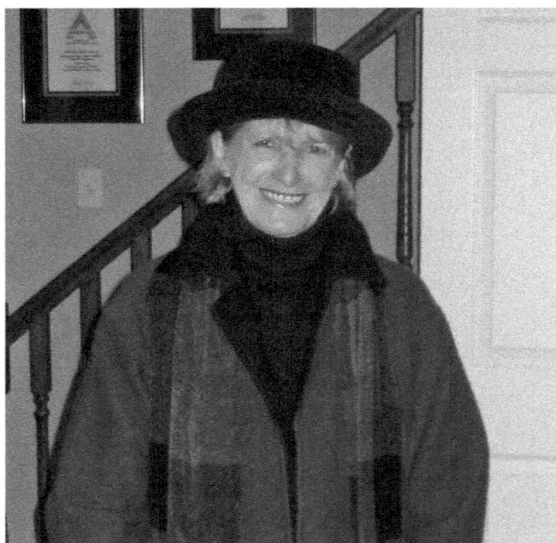

Afterword

In the ten years that passed between my mother's death and the release of this memoir, I have approached each day with the certainty that both my mother and father remain with me always. My mother's red and white roses, and my father's stargazer lilies, appear whenever I most need them. The examples my parents set and the lessons they taught guide every aspect of my life, both in terms of how I live it and what I try to accomplish.

And to a large degree, I will always see and judge myself through my mother's eyes, and be the better for it.

Read the Award-Winning Alzheimer's Memoir

TENTH ANNIVERSARY EDITION

STANDING TALL

A Daughter's
Gift

The mind forgets. The soul remembers.

JACQUI TAM

For more information, visit:
www.icebergpublishing.com

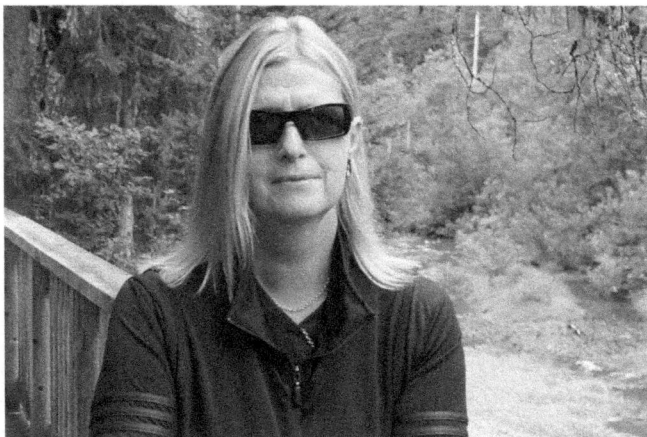

About the Author

Jacqui Tam is an award-winning communications professional, author, and publisher. An intensely proud Newfoundlander, she has lived and worked in eastern, central and western Canada. Her career has taken her to the executive level in the higher education sector, with involvement in a variety of national and international organizations.

Most of her writing is non-fiction.

And mostly she still listens more than she talks.

Find Jacqui Tam on social media at @JTam_Iceberg
and read her blog at www.icebergpublishing.com.

www.ingramcontent.com/pod-product-compliance
Lightning Source LLC
Chambersburg PA
CBHW032114280326
41933CB00009B/834